How To Reduce Pot Belly

A Comprehensive Guide to Shedding Belly Fat and Regaining Your Health

Janet Jones

Janet Jones

Table of Contents

Introduction

Mark came to a fork in the road in a peaceful residential area. His self-esteem was at an all-time low since he had battled his pot belly for years.

He stumbled across a book that would transform his life one day while perusing a nearby bookshop.

This modest book ended up becoming Mark's compass. Its pages were jam-packed with useful information, from explaining the physics behind belly fat to offering in-depth fitness plans and dietary suggestions. Mark applied the lessons from the book, changing his diet to include healthful foods and resolving to engage in regular exercise.

But the focus on mindfulness and motivation was what set this book apart. It taught Mark to appreciate his progress and to stay inspired in the face of adversity. He found encouragement in the book's stress-reduction tips, and soon his transition to a healthy lifestyle became a way of life.

Mark's pot belly started to become smaller over time, but more significantly, his confidence increased. He had lost weight thanks to the book's advice and wisdom, but it had also changed his perspective. Mark served as evidence that progress could be made one page at a time.

Chapter 1

The Science of Belly Fat

Understanding the Problem

The first and most important step in minimizing a pot belly is understanding the issue. Beyond being unsightly, a pot belly, which is often brought on by too much visceral fat, carries health dangers.

It raises your chance of developing diabetes, heart disease, and other chronic illnesses. Understanding the underlying causes, such as poor food choices, a sedentary lifestyle, and hormone imbalances, is necessary to properly treat it.

Individuals are inspired to make significant behavioral adjustments and emphasize leading healthier, more active lives when they realize that a pot belly is more than simply a cosmetic worry.

Establishing Your Goals

The next crucial step in getting rid of a pot belly is setting your objectives. Setting direction and motivational objectives that are clear and doable.

Think about your goals, whether they be to lose a specific amount of weight, trim down your waist, or become more physically active. Make sure your objectives are precise, quantifiable, and time-limited. For instance, set a goal to reduce your waistline by 2 inches in three months.

Setting these goals helps you stay motivated and focused by enabling you to monitor your progress and recognize your accomplishments as you go, making the journey to a healthy one more enjoyable and doable.

Why Does Pot Belly Occur?

Various underlying factors may contribute to pot belly or abdominal obesity:

1. Poor Diet: Consuming too many calories, particularly from processed foods and sugary beverages, promotes the development of belly fat.

2. Insufficient Exercise: Sedentary behavior slows metabolism and promotes fat accumulation, which includes belly fat.

3. Genetics: The distribution of body fat may be influenced by genetics, making certain people more likely to have a pot belly.

4. Hormonal Changes: Abdominal fat growth may result from hormonal abnormalities such as high cortisol levels (a stress hormone) or insulin resistance.

5. Aging: As individuals become older, their metabolisms tend to slow down, which might increase the likelihood that belly fat will collect.

6. Stress: Due to elevated cortisol levels, long-term stress may cause overeating and result in belly weight gain.

7. Insufficient Sleep: Belly fat may develop as a result of disturbed hormone rhythms that control hunger and metabolism.

8. Drinking Alcohol: Alcoholism in excess may cause fat to accumulate in the abdomen, a condition known as "beer belly."

9. Medical Illnesses: Abdominal obesity may be brought on by certain medical illnesses including polycystic ovarian syndrome (PCOS) or Cushing's syndrome.

Understanding these factors is crucial for tackling the source of the issue and creating successful pot belly-reducing techniques.

Various Forms of Belly Fat

Based on its location and features, belly fat may be divided into many types:

1. Subcutaneous Fat: When the belly is squeezed, this fat—which is located right under the skin—appears squishy and jiggly. Although extra subcutaneous fat may lead to a pot belly, visceral fat is more hazardous to health.

2. Visceral Fat: Deeper inside the abdominal cavity, visceral fat surrounds important organs including the liver, pancreas, and intestines. Visceral fat that is too much is significantly linked to health concerns such as metabolic syndrome, diabetes, and heart disease.

3. Central Obesity: Central obesity, often referred to as android obesity, is characterized by an abundance of fat, mostly in the abdomen region. It often entails an "apple-shaped" physique and a greater risk of health problems.

4. Lower Belly Fat: It might be difficult to work against this kind of fat since it likes to collect in the lower abdomen area. It often causes anxiety for both hygienic and cosmetic reasons.

5. Fat In The Upper Belly: Just below the ribs, in the upper abdominal region, there is a concentration of belly fat. Health hazards may also be connected to it, particularly when visceral fat is present.

It's crucial to comprehend the many forms of belly fat since they may react differently to dietary, physical activity, and lifestyle modifications. For bettering general health and lowering the risk of chronic illnesses,

visceral fat reduction in particular is
essential.

Chapter 2

The Importance of Diet

By regulating calorie intake, encouraging fat reduction, and maintaining hormonal balance, diet plays a crucial part in minimizing pot belly. Unwanted belly fat may be lost with a well-balanced diet full of whole foods, fiber, lean proteins, and healthy fats. For pot belly reduction to be successful, processed and sugary meals must be avoided.

Good Eating Practices for Reducing Pot Belly

1. Balanced Meals: Eat meals that are well-balanced and include lean protein, whole grains, fruits, veggies, and healthy fats. This gives you vital nutrients and prolongs your feeling of fullness.

2. Portion Control: Watch the sizes of your portions to prevent overeating. Use smaller plates and be mindful of your portion sizes.

3. Foods High in Fiber: Include foods rich in fiber, such as whole grains, legumes, and veggies. Fiber helps with digestion and appetite regulation.

4. Limit Foods High In Sugar: Cut down on processed food, sweetened beverages, and sweets. Sugar consumption in excess might increase abdominal fat.

5. Hydration: Drink plenty of water to stay hydrated. Sometimes, hunger and thirst are confused.

6. Protein Intake: Include lean protein sources in your diet to assist muscle building and regulate hunger, such as chicken, fish, tofu, and beans.

7. Suitable Fats: Choose healthy fats from sources like avocados, almonds, and olive oil. They support general health and satiety.

8. Regular Meals: Never miss a meal. To keep blood sugar levels constant and avoid overeating, eat often.

9. Mindful Consumption: Eat mindfully, enjoying each mouthful, and free of interruptions. Thus, mindless munching may be avoided.

10. Meal Planning: Make healthier options easily accessible by planning meals and snacks.

Adopting these healthy eating practices may considerably help with weight loss and general well-being.

Avoiding Certain Foods to Reduce Pot Belly

1. Sugary Drinks: Fruit juices, energy drinks, sweetened teas, and sugary sodas should all be avoided or limited. These provide a lot of empty calories and might make you gain weight.

2. Foods That Have Been Processed: Reduce consumption of sugary cereals, chips, and processed snacks. They often include too much salt and trans fats.

3. Excessive Sugar: Avoid eating too much sugar by limiting your intake of sweets, pastries, and candy. Sugar consumption in excess might increase abdominal fat.

4. Trans Fats: Steer clear of items containing trans fats, including numerous packaged snacks and fried fast food. They are linked to heart disease and weight gain.

5. Pastries and White Bread: White bread and pastries, which are rich in refined carbs, should be substituted with whole-grain choices.

6. Alcohol: Consume alcohol in moderation since excessive alcohol use may result in abdominal weight gain, sometimes known as a "beer belly."

7. Processed Meats: Reduce your intake of highly processed meats like sausages, bacon, and deli meats since they often include dangerous additives.

8. Sweetened Additives: Be careful when using condiments that may include a lot of added sugar, such as ketchup and barbecue sauce.

9. Fast Food: Due to its high calorie, fat, and sugar content, limit your intake of fast food.

10. Synthetic Sweeteners: Artificial sweeteners may interfere with the control of appetite, according to certain research, which might result in overeating.

You may successfully minimize pot belly and enhance your general health by avoiding these items and putting an emphasis on a balanced, whole-foods-based diet.

Putting Together a Balanced Diet Plan for Pot Belly Reduction

1. Assess Your Current Diet: Start by assessing your present eating patterns and pinpointing what needs to change.

2. Set Realistic Goals: Specify reachable objectives for decreasing the pot belly, such as precise weight loss goals or measures of the waist.

3. Whole Foods: Use entire, unprocessed foods like fruits, vegetables, whole grains, lean meats, and healthy fats as the foundation of your diet.

4. Portion Control: Portion control is important to prevent overeating. Measure portions and use smaller plates.

5. Frequent Meals: To maintain stable blood sugar levels and avoid excessive hunger, have frequent, balanced meals.

6. Protein: To boost muscle building and curb hunger, include lean protein foods including chicken, fish, tofu, beans, and lentils.

7. Foods High in Fiber: It helps with digestion and encourages fullness, giving fiber-rich meals like vegetables, whole grains, and legumes priority.

8. Healthy Fats: Pick healthy fats from sources like avocados, almonds, seeds, and olive oil. These fats promote satiety and general wellness.

9. Limit Sugars: Reduce additional sugars in your diet by staying away from sugary beverages, sweets, and snacks.

10. Hydroponics: Drink plenty of water throughout the day to be appropriately hydrated since hunger and thirst may often be confused.

11. Plan your Meal: Plan your meals and snacks ahead of time to ensure that you have access to nutrient-dense selections.

12. Varieties: To ensure you obtain a variety of nutrients, include a variety of foods in your diet.

13. Mindful Eating: Practice mindful eating by taking your time with each mouthful, eating without interruptions, and paying attention to your body's hunger and fullness signs.

Always keep in mind that developing a balanced food plan entails making long-lasting, enduring adjustments. It's important to improve general health and well-being in addition to pot belly reduction.

Chapter 3

Effective Exercises

Cardio activities (like jogging or cycling), strength training (like planks and squats), and core exercises (like crunches and leg lifts) are all good ways to lose belly fat. Combining these exercises promotes muscular growth and fat loss.

Cardio Exercises to Reduce Pot Belly

Exercises that increase the heart rate and blood flow are known as cardiovascular exercises, sometimes known as cardio or aerobic workouts.

Here are some heart-healthy workouts to try:

1. **Running**: Running is a high-intensity aerobic exercise that works for many muscle groups and effectively burns calories, whether it is done outside or on a treadmill.

2. **Cycling:** Biking is a low-impact aerobic activity that is easy on the joints and may help reduce tummy fat.

3. **Swimming:** Swimming offers a total-body exercise that not only helps you lose weight but also strengthens your core and enhances your fitness level.

4. **Quickly Moving:** Brisk walking is a simple yet effective activity that increases heart rate and promotes fat reduction.

5. **Jumping Rope:** Jumping rope is a great aerobic exercise since it raises your heart rate quickly and effectively, which helps you burn calories.

6. Dancing: In addition to being fun, dancing to your favorite music may help you lose weight and enhance cardiovascular health.

7. High-Intensity Interval Training (HIIT): Short bursts of intensive activity are interspersed with quick rest intervals during HIIT exercises. They may burn fat, especially belly fat, quite effectively.

8. Stair Climbing: Climbing steps or utilizing a stair climber machine works on your lower body and core while also getting your heart rate up.

9. Elliptical Exerciser: This low-impact exercise equipment works the whole body and is excellent for those with joint problems.

10. Rowing: Rowing machines help you burn calories while strengthening your core and upper body. They also improve your cardiovascular health.

Aim for at least 150 minutes of moderate-intensity cardio activity or 75 minutes of vigorous-intensity cardio exercise per week, together with a balanced diet and other specialized workouts, to successfully decrease pot belly.

Strength Training for Pot Belly Reduction

Resistance training sometimes referred to as strength training, is a crucial part of any fitness program that works to get rid of the muffin top. It entails engaging in physical activity that puts your muscles up against opposition.

The following is a description of several important strength training exercises:

1. Planks: A core-strengthening exercise called a plank requires you to maintain a push-up posture with your arms or forearms. The abdominal muscles are strengthened and toned as a result.

2. Squats: Squats target the glutes, hamstrings, and quadriceps muscles in your lower body. For stability, they also make your core work.

3. Push-Ups: Push-ups exercise the triceps, shoulders, and chest. They are largely an upper body workout, but they also work the core to keep the body upright.

4. Leggings: Targeting your legs' muscles, such as the quadriceps, hamstrings, and glutes, is made easy with lunges. For balance, they also include your core.

5. Deadlifting: Your hamstrings, glutes, and lower back are the main muscles that are used during a deadlift. They work a variety of muscle groups since they are complex exercises.

6. Russian Twists: The oblique muscles on the sides of your abdomen are strengthened by this workout. Your torso must be twisted while you are carrying a weight or medicine ball.

7. Leg Raising: Leg raises are a good exercise to focus on the lower abdominal muscles. Laying on your back, raise your legs toward the ceiling while maintaining a strong core.

8. Kettlebell Swings: Kettlebell swings exercise the lower back, glutes, and hamstrings as well as the complete posterior chain. For stability, they also engage the core.

9. Bent-Over Rows: Bent-over rows target the biceps and upper back muscles.

They aid in strengthening the upper body and enhancing posture.

10. Bicep Curls Using Dumbbells: This workout targets only the biceps, which helps the arm muscles become toned and stronger.

Strength training helps people lose total fat, particularly belly fat, while also enhancing muscle growth and metabolism. Target various muscle groups using a range of these exercises to develop a well-rounded strength training regimen. For best results, try to undertake strength training activities two to three times each week.

Chapter 4

Lifestyle Changes

Making healthy choices in your lifestyle, such as managing your stress, eating a balanced diet, getting enough sleep, and being hydrated, may help you lose weight. These adjustments support long-term weight reduction and general well-being.

Stress Management For Reducing Pot Belly

The key to decreasing pot belly is stress reduction. Due to increased cortisol production, elevated stress levels may cause weight gain, especially in the abdomen region.

Here are some tips for handling stress well:

1. Exercise Regularly: Regular exercise helps to lower stress hormones and encourage relaxation. Some suggestions include yoga, meditation, or deep breathing techniques.

3. Mindful Exercise: Practice mindfulness exercises and meditation to build a state of calm and lessen emotional eating brought on by stress.

4. Time Management: Create a set timetable for the day to reduce stress brought on by hurried tasks or missed deadlines.

5. Healthy Coping Strategies: Swap out negative coping strategies like emotional eating with constructive ones like keeping a diary, speaking with a friend, or partaking in a beloved pastime.

6. Limit Stimulants: Limit coffee and alcohol intake since too much of either may worsen stress and interfere with sleep.

7. Ask For Help: When stress gets unbearable, ask for help by contacting friends, family, or a mental health professional. Your emotional weight may be less if you share your worries.

8. Relaxation Techniques: Explore relaxing techniques like progressive muscle relaxation or aromatherapy to decompress and lessen tension.

9. Balanced Diet: Maintain a balanced diet full of nutrient-rich foods to enhance your ability to cope with stress and your general well-being.

10. Reduce Screen Time: particularly before night, and avoid news or social media that might cause stress.

You may reduce cortisol levels, avoid stress-related weight gain, and contribute to a better lifestyle overall by actively managing your stress using these techniques. This will help you lose weight and get rid of your pot belly.

Quality Sleep to Reduce Pot Belly

To lose belly fat, getting enough sleep is essential since it has a direct impact on the hormones that control appetite and metabolism.

The following tips can help you obtain the restorative sleep you need to lose weight effectively:

1. **Consistent Routine:** Maintain a consistent routine by going to bed and getting up at the same times every day, even on weekends.

2. **Sleep Environment:** A cold, calm, and dark room can help you get a good night's sleep. Purchase supportive pillows and a mattress.

3. Limiting Screen Time: This is important since the blue light from devices like phones, TVs, and laptops may interfere with sleep.

4. Relaxation Techniques: Practice relaxation techniques before going to bed to settle your thoughts, such as deep breathing, meditation, or light stretching.

5. Limit Coffee And Alcohol Intake: since these substances may impair the quality of your sleep.

6. Regular Physical Exercise: Take part in regular physical exercise, but stay away from demanding workouts just before night.

7. Light Exposure: Get exposure to natural light throughout the day to optimize your sleep-wake habits and regulate your body's internal clock.

8. Avoid Heavy Meals: Avoid consuming a lot of food soon before bed. Choose a light snack if necessary.

9. Limiting Fluid Consumption: It can help you avoid waking up in the middle of the night to use the bathroom.

10. Manage Stress: Practice mindfulness and relaxation strategies to lessen worry, which may interfere with sleep.

Making regular sleep a priority promotes hormonal balance, lessens food cravings, and improves your body's capacity to burn fat, all of which eventually help you lose weight and get rid of your muffin top.

Hydration to Reduce Pot Belly

A key component of reducing abdominal fat and improving general health is staying well hydrated.

Why staying hydrated is important and methods to do so are as follows:

1. **Appetite Management:** Adequate water may aid with appetite management. Sometimes the body conflates hunger with thirst, which results in unneeded eating.

2. **Digestion:** Water helps with digestion and avoids constipation, ensuring that your body breaks down food properly.

3. **Metabolism:** Hydration boosts metabolism, which enables your body to burn calories more efficiently.

4. **Fluid Equilibrium:** Hydration preserves the body's fluid equilibrium, which is essential for general health and weight control.

Tips To Remain Hydrated:

- **Drink Water Regularly:** Although individual requirements may vary, aim to consume at least eight 8-ounce glasses (or around 2 liters) of water each day.

- **Check The Color Of Your Urine:** It should be a light yellow. Urine that is dark yellow or amber may be a sign of dehydration.

- **Hydrate Before Meals:** Before meals, drink a glass of water to help regulate your appetite and prevent overeating.

- **Have a Water Bottle:** To promote frequent sips, have a reusable water bottle with you at all times.

- **Incorporate Hydrating Meals:** For increased hydration, eat water-rich meals such as fruits and vegetables (such as lettuce and celery).

- **Limit Sugary Drinks:** Steer clear of sweetened drinks like soda, which may result in a surplus of calories consumed and weight gain.

Your quest to lose belly fat and maintain a healthy body composition includes a balanced diet, an active lifestyle, and proper hydration.

Chapter 5

The Importance of Portion Control

Portion management is essential for reducing pot belly since it guards against overeating, regulates calorie intake, and aids in weight loss. You may develop a sustainable, balanced diet that helps you reach and maintain a healthy weight by controlling portion sizes.

Mindful Eating to Reduce Pot Belly

The practice of mindful eating entails being completely present during the whole eating process, including the tastes, textures, and experiences.

Encouraging healthy eating choices may considerably help with pot belly reduction:

1. Awareness: Mindful eating promotes awareness of what and why you eat, assisting you in differentiating between emotional and physical hunger cues.

2. Portion Management: It improves attention to your body's hunger and fullness signals, avoiding overeating and encouraging portion management.

3. Enjoyment: By taking your time to enjoy every mouthful, you're more likely to enjoy the tastes of nutrient-dense meals, which makes them a more fulfilling option.

4. Reduced Stress Eating: Stress-related emotional eating, which may increase belly fat, can be reduced with mindful eating.

5. Improved Digestion: Eating slowly and deliberately improves digestion, which lowers the risk of bloating and discomfort.

To eat mindfully, concentrate on chewing your meal properly and paying attention to your body's fullness cues while avoiding any outside distractions. By using this mindful eating strategy, you may better control your diet and help reduce your belly fat.

The Plate Approach

The Plate Method is a method of balanced eating that is practical and may be especially beneficial in reducing abdominal fat.

This is how it goes:

1. Divide Your Plate: Divide your plate into pieces in your head as follows:

- Non-starchy vegetables like leafy greens, broccoli, or peppers should make about half of the meal. These are high in fiber and minerals yet low in calories.

- Lean protein sources like chicken, fish, tofu, or beans should make up one-fourth of the dish.

- Whole grains or starchy vegetables like brown rice, quinoa, or sweet potatoes may take up the remaining quarter of the plate.

2. Add Fruits: A modest amount of fruit or a fruit salad might be added as a side dish or dessert.

3. Healthy Fats: A source of healthy fats in your diet by adding olive oil to veggies or a handful of almonds as a snack.

4. Portion Awareness: The Plate Method promotes portion management by visibly separating your plate, which makes it simpler to keep track of calorie consumption.

5. Balanced Nutrition: This strategy guarantees a balance of necessary nutrients while limiting portion sizes, which is vital for reducing pot belly.

6. Fiber-Focused: Focusing on veggies and whole grains helps you naturally consume more fiber, which helps you feel fuller and maintain good digestive health.

7. Awareness: Water or other hydrating liquids should be consumed with meals to aid digestion and curb hunger.

The Plate Method promotes a balanced diet that helps reduce belly fat, encourages mindful eating, and makes meal planning easier. It's an effective tool for obtaining and maintaining a healthy weight, portion management, and body composition.

Chapter 6

Tracking Your Progress

Monitoring your progress can help you remain motivated and make the necessary corrections as you work to lose that pot belly.

Establishing Milestones

Setting Pot Belly Reduction Milestones

A smart strategy for reaching your pot belly reduction objectives is to set milestones. These intermediate goals enable you to track your progress and maintain motivation.

How to establish milestones is as follows:

1. **Defined Goals:** Establish clear objectives for what you wish to accomplish. For instance, be specific about how much weight or belly fat you intend to shed.

2. Break It Down: Break your main objective down into smaller, more doable benchmarks. These might occur once a month or every three months.

3. Use Measurable Metrics: Use quantitative metrics to ensure that your accomplishments can be monitored and measured. Weight, waist size, and body fat percentage are a few examples.

4. Establish A Timeline: Give each milestone an appropriate time limit. Setting realistic deadlines will keep you dedicated and focused.

5. Celebrate Your Successes: Give Yourself a Treat When You Reach A Milestone. Honoring accomplishments strengthens your resolve and raises your spirits.

6. Adjust as Needed: Be adaptable and prepared to change your goals if required. Diet and exercise may have different effects on your body.

7. Stay Consistent: Achieving objectives requires consistency. Maintain a strict diet and workout schedule.

8. Accountability: Share your achievements with a friend, a member of your family, or a fitness partner who can provide motivation and hold you accountable.

Typical Milestones

- 5 pounds should be lost in the first month.

- In two months, reduce waist size by one inch.

- Continue a consistent workout schedule for three months.

- Attain a predetermined body fat percentage in less than six months.

Setting goals for pot belly reduction helps you feel accomplished as you complete each one and makes the process more doable. It aids in your continued motivation and dedication to your long-term objective.

Measuring Pot Belly Reduction Success

Examining many indications of weight is necessary to determine the effectiveness of pot belly reduction.

Here are some crucial criteria to take into account while gauging your progress:

1. **Waist Circumference:** Waist circumference decrease is often a more precise indicator of pot belly reduction than total weight.

2. Body Fat Percentage: Monitoring changes in body fat percentage gives you information about changes in your body's composition.

3. Health Indicators: Monitor health indicators that may indicate increased health, which include blood pressure, cholesterol levels, and blood sugar.

4. Clothes Fitting: Examine how your clothing fits to see if you can easily fit into lower sizes.

5. Energy Levels: Check to see whether you have more vigor and endurance for everyday tasks and exercises.

6. Physical Fitness: Keep track of your progress in terms of your strength, stamina, and flexibility.

7. Nutritional Habits: Examine your nutritional habits, such as if you have less desire for harmful meals and whether you practice mindful eating.

8. Measurements Of Emotional Well-being: This includes lower levels of stress, better moods, and higher levels of self-esteem.

9. Consistency: Evaluate your capacity to lead a healthy lifestyle over time with consistency.

10. Quality of Life: Consider enhancements to your general quality of life, such as greater sleep, fewer stomach problems, and improved mobility.

Keep in mind that losing abdominal fat is much more than just a weight. A holistic approach is used in the pursuit of greater health and well-being.

You may better comprehend your progress and overall accomplishments by gauging success using a mix of these markers.

Chapter 7

Conclusion

For a healthier, happier self, embrace a balanced diet, regular exercise, mindfulness, and tenacity in your quest to lose the pot belly.

Here is a summary of methods to lose abdominal fat:

1. Balanced Nutrition: Lean meats, fruits, vegetables, and healthy fats should all be included in a diet that is balanced and consists of complete, unprocessed foods. Portion management should also be practiced.

2. Cardio Workouts: To burn calories and decrease total body fat, including belly fat, include cardiovascular workouts like jogging, cycling, or swimming.

3. Strength Training: Include strength training to develop lean muscle, speed up metabolism, and promote a toned abdomen.

4. Core Exercises: Exercise your core to develop your abdominal muscles and correct your posture.

5. Mindful Eating: To be aware of hunger signals, prevent emotional eating, and relish each meal, engage in mindful eating.

6. The Plate Method: When portioning your meals, use the Plate Method to emphasize veggies, lean meats, and nutritious grains.

7. Hydration: Water consumption all day long can help you stay hydrated, which will help you manage your hunger and assist your metabolism.

8. Stress Reduction: To avoid stress-related weight gain, manage your stress using strategies like exercise, meditation, and enough sleep.

9. Quality Sleep: Prioritize getting great sleep to balance hormones, restrain hunger, and aid in weight reduction.

10. Portion Control: Control portion sizes to prevent overeating and efficiently control calorie intake.

11. Tracking Progress: To keep on track, take measurements of your waist and your level of fitness.

12. Setting Milestones: To monitor your progress toward reducing your pot belly, set precise, quantifiable, and time-bound objectives.

13. Measuring Success: Measure success using a variety of indicators, such as waist size, body fat percentage, health indicators, garment fit, and general well-being.

14. Consistency: Maintaining consistency in your healthy behaviors over time can help you attain long-lasting outcomes.

You may work towards minimizing pot belly and enhancing your general health and fitness by putting these techniques into practice regularly and individualizing them to meet your requirements.

Keep in mind that perseverance and commitment are essential for long-term success.

Adopting a Healthier Way of Life

Changing to a healthy lifestyle requires a dedication to one's total well-being, not just to weight loss.

This is how:

1. Nutrition: Make thoughtful decisions about your diet by choosing healthy foods, sensible serving sizes, and mindful eating.

2. Exercise: Make it a lifetime habit to move your body, concentrating on cardio, strength, and core workouts.

3. Mindfulness: For long-lasting transformation, cultivate awareness of diet, stress, and self-care.

4. Sleep: Prioritize restful sleep to support your body's physiological functions.

5. Stress Management: Building resilience against life's hardships via relaxation and emotional equilibrium is known as stress management.

6. Consistency: It's a marathon, not a sprint, as you travel. Remain dedicated to being healthy.

7. Self-Care: Feed your body and mind with love, tolerance, and compassion for yourself.

8. Lifelong Learning: Continue to learn and modify your way of life as you advance.

Adopting these concepts helps you lose weight while promoting long-term health, happiness, and energy.

Bonus: Healthy Recipes

Incorporating a variety of healthy recipes into your meal planning can be a powerful strategy for pot belly reduction, as it combines balanced nutrition with flavorful, satisfying dishes that support your goals and long-term well-being.

Nutritious Meal Ideas

1. Grilled Chicken Salad
Description: Grilled chicken breast on a bed of mixed greens with cherry tomatoes, cucumber, and a balsamic vinaigrette.
Calories: Approximately 350 calories per serving.
Key Info: High in protein, fiber, and essential vitamins.

2. Quinoa and Vegetable Stir-Fry
Description: Stir-fry quinoa with colorful vegetables and a light soy-ginger sauce.

Calories: Approximately 400 calories per serving.

Key Info: Packed with protein, fiber, and various nutrients.

3. Lentil and Vegetable Soup

Description: Hearty soup with lentils, carrots, celery, and spices in a vegetable broth.

Calories: Approximately 250 calories per serving.

Key Info: High in fiber, plant-based protein, and low in fat.

4. Baked Salmon with Asparagus

Description: Oven-baked salmon filet seasoned with lemon and herbs, served with roasted asparagus.

Calories: Approximately 350 calories per serving.

Key Info: Rich in omega-3 fatty acids, lean protein, and antioxidants.

5. Spinach and Mushroom Omelette

Description: Fluffy omelette filled with sautéed spinach, mushrooms, and a sprinkle of low-fat cheese.

Calories: Approximately 300 calories per serving.

Key Info: High in protein, vitamins, and minerals.

6. Chickpea and Vegetable Curry

Description: Flavorful curry with chickpeas, assorted vegetables, and aromatic spices served with brown rice.

Calories: Approximately 400 calories per serving.

Key Info: Rich in plant-based protein, fiber, and antioxidants.

7. Turkey and Avocado Wrap

Description: Whole-grain wrap filled with lean turkey, sliced avocado, lettuce, and a touch of mustard.

Calories: Approximately 350 calories per serving.

Key Info: Good source of protein, healthy fats, and fiber.

8. Greek Yogurt Parfait

Description: Layer Greek yogurt with fresh berries, granola, and a drizzle of honey.

Calories: Approximately 250 calories per serving.

Key Info: High in protein, probiotics, and antioxidants.

9. Sweet Potato and Black Bean Bowl

Description: Roasted sweet potatoes and black beans, topped with salsa, avocado, and a dollop of Greek yogurt.

Calories: Approximately 400 calories per serving.

Key Info: Packed with fiber, plant-based protein, and vitamins.

10. Tofu and Vegetable Stir-Fry

Description: Stir-fry tofu with a colorful medley of vegetables and a savory stir-fry sauce, served over brown rice.

Calories: Approximately 350 calories per serving.

Key Info: High in plant-based protein, fiber, and low in saturated fat.

These nutritious meal ideas provide a variety of flavors and nutrients while keeping calories in check, making them excellent choices for a balanced and health-conscious meal.